PART 2

HEALTHY

AND

POISON

FOOD COMBINATIONS

Health wellness

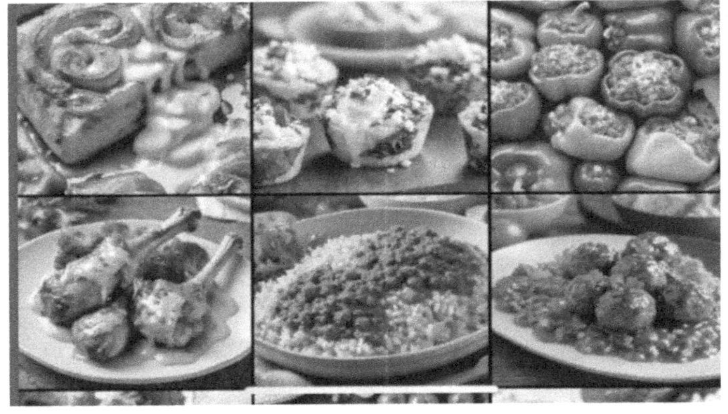

Introduction

Once upon a time, in a quaint town nestled between rolling hills, lived a man named Oliver. Known for his adventurous palate, Oliver took pride in experimenting with unique food combinations. One fateful day, he decided to create a dish that blended flavors in ways that had never been attempted before.

In his small kitchen, Oliver gathered an assortment of ingredients: spicy peppers, sweet fruits, rich cheeses, and exotic spices. With unwavering confidence, he concocted a dish that seemed like a masterpiece on his taste buds. Ignoring traditional culinary wisdom, he devoured the unconventional fusion.

As the hours passed, Oliver began to feel an unsettling discomfort in his stomach. The once vibrant hues of the dish now seemed like a harbinger of his impending doom. Ignoring the warning signs, he dismissed the discomfort as mere indigestion.

However, the combination of incompatible ingredients took a toll on his digestive system. Agony gripped him, and his condition worsened rapidly. Panicking, Oliver sought medical attention, but it was too late. The doctors struggled to understand the unusual mix of elements wreaking havoc inside him.

With regret and sorrow, Oliver succumbed to the consequences of his daring culinary experiment. The town mourned the loss of their adventurous food enthusiast, a cautionary tale echoing through the streets about the importance of respecting the delicate balance of flavors in the pursuit of gastronomic pleasure.

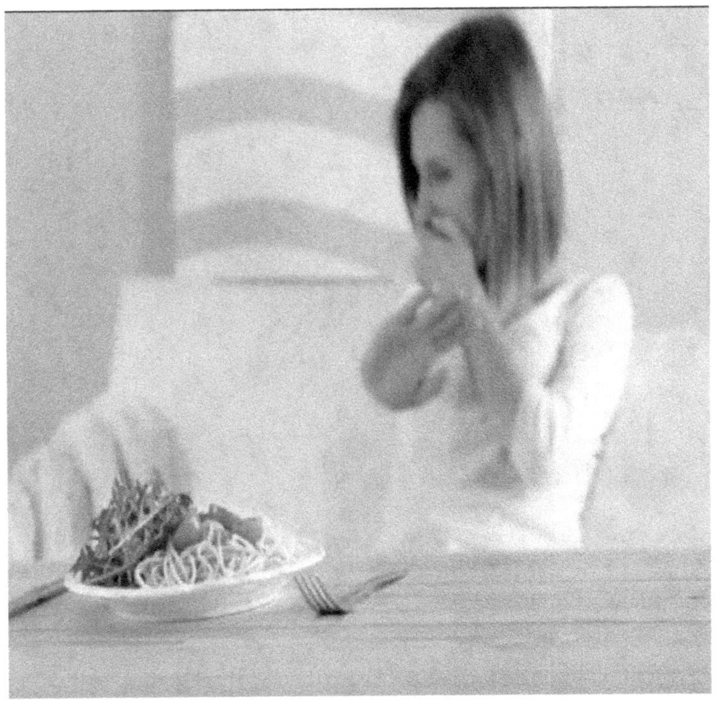

TABLE OF CONTENTS

Introduction

CHAPTER 1 :Culinary Harmony

Creating Flavorful and Nutrient-Rich Meals

Exploring Global Cuisine for Inspired Combinations

CHAPTER 2 :Special Considerations

Food Combinations for Specific Diets (e.g., Vegan, Paleo)

Tailoring Combinations for Dietary Restrictions

CHAPTER 3 :Digestive Health

Promoting Gut Health through Smart Food Choices

Foods that Aid Digestion

CHAPTER 4:Recipes and Practical Examples

Breakfast Ideas for Delicious Food Combinations

Lunch and Dinner Combinations

Snack Options

CHAPTER 5:Summary of Key Principle

Incorporating Food Combinations into Daily

Life

CHAPTER 1 :Culinary Harmony

Culinary Harmony is a concept that revolves around the seamless integration of diverse flavors, textures, and cooking techniques to create a balanced and harmonious culinary experience. It goes beyond mere recipe execution, emphasizing a thoughtful combination of ingredients that complement each other in taste and nutritional value.

In the world of Culinary Harmony, chefs strive to achieve a symphony of flavors by understanding the principles of taste, such as sweet, salty, sour, bitter, and umami. By skillfully blending these elements, they create dishes that tantalize the palate and leave a lasting impression on diners.

This culinary philosophy also extends to the aesthetic presentation of dishes, considering color, texture, and arrangement on the plate. The goal is to engage not only the sense of taste but also sight, enhancing the overall dining experience.

Culinary Harmony emphasizes the use of fresh, seasonal ingredients to capture the essence of each component at its peak. It encourages chefs to explore local and global cuisines, drawing inspiration from various culinary traditions to craft innovative and well-balanced menus.

Technological advancements and modern cooking techniques play a role in achieving Culinary Harmony, allowing chefs to experiment with molecular gastronomy, sous-vide cooking, and other methods that enhance precision and control over the cooking process.

Culinary education and training are vital aspects of embracing this concept, as chefs learn to master the art of flavor pairing, ingredient sourcing, and creative expression in the kitchen. It fosters a mindset that values not only the final dish but also the journey of crafting it.

Restaurants and culinary establishments that embrace Culinary Harmony often focus on sustainability and ethical sourcing practices. They aim to create a positive impact on both the environment and the communities they serve, promoting a holistic approach to food preparation and consumption.

In conclusion, Culinary Harmony is a holistic approach to cooking that goes beyond the technical aspects of culinary arts. It encompasses a deep understanding of flavors, a creative exploration of ingredients, and a commitment to sustainability, resulting in a dining experience that is not only delicious but also harmonious in every sense.

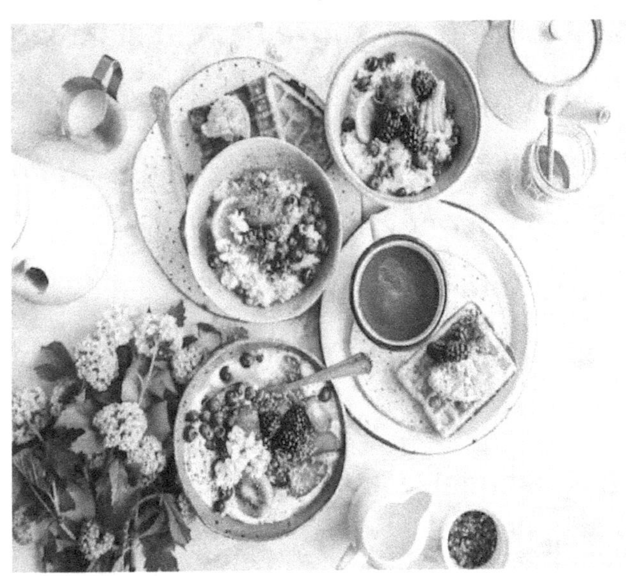

Creating flavorful and nutrient-rich meals is a delightful journey that involves a thoughtful selection of ingredients, creative cooking techniques, and an understanding of nutritional balance. Here's a comprehensive guide to help you embark on this culinary adventure:

Ingredient Selection:

- **Fresh Produce**: Opt for a variety of colorful fruits and vegetables, as they provide essential vitamins, minerals, and antioxidants.

- **Lean Proteins**: Include sources like poultry, fish, beans, and tofu for protein without excessive saturated fats.

- **Whole Grains**: Choose whole grains like quinoa, brown rice, and oats for added fiber, promoting digestive health.

- **Healthy Fats**: Incorporate sources like avocados, nuts, and olive oil for heart-healthy fats and improved satiety.

Flavor Enhancement:

- **Herbs and Spices**: Experiment with herbs like basil, thyme, and spices like cumin, paprika to add depth without extra calories.

- **Citrus Zest**: Grate citrus peels for a burst of flavor without added sodium.

- **Garlic and Onions**: These aromatic ingredients bring a savory note to dishes without relying on excessive salt or sugar.

Cooking Techniques:

- **Grilling and Roasting**: Enhance flavors by grilling or roasting vegetables and proteins, creating a caramelized exterior.

- **Sauteing**: Use minimal oil when sautéing to preserve nutrients and create a rich flavor profile.

- **Steaming**: Retain nutrients by steaming vegetables, fish, or poultry, ensuring a vibrant color and crisp texture.

Nutritional Balance:

- **Protein-Packed Meals**: Include a balance of protein, carbohydrates, and healthy fats to promote sustained energy and muscle health.

- **Portion Control**: Maintain a balance in portion sizes to avoid overconsumption while still satisfying your appetite.

- **Colorful Plates**: Aim for a diverse color palette on your plate, indicating a variety of nutrients.

Meal Planning and Preparation:

- **Weekly Planning**: Plan your meals for the week, incorporating a mix of proteins, vegetables, and grains to ensure a well-rounded diet.

- **Batch Cooking**: Save time and ensure nutritious meals by preparing larger batches and storing portions for later consumption.

Mindful Eating:

- **Savoring Each Bite**: Pay attention to the taste, texture, and aroma of your food to foster a mindful eating experience.

- **Listening to Hunger Cues**: Tune in to your body's hunger and fullness signals, promoting a healthy relationship with food.

Hydration:

- **Water Infusion**: Add natural flavors to your water by infusing it with fruits, herbs, or cucumber, encouraging proper hydration.

- **Limit Sugary Drinks**: Minimize the intake of sugary beverages, opting for water, herbal teas, or infused water instead. By combining these principles, you'll not only create meals bursting with flavor but also provide your body with a diverse range of essential nutrients for overall well-being. Enjoy the journey of crafting delicious and nutritionally-rich dishes that contribute to a healthier lifestyle.

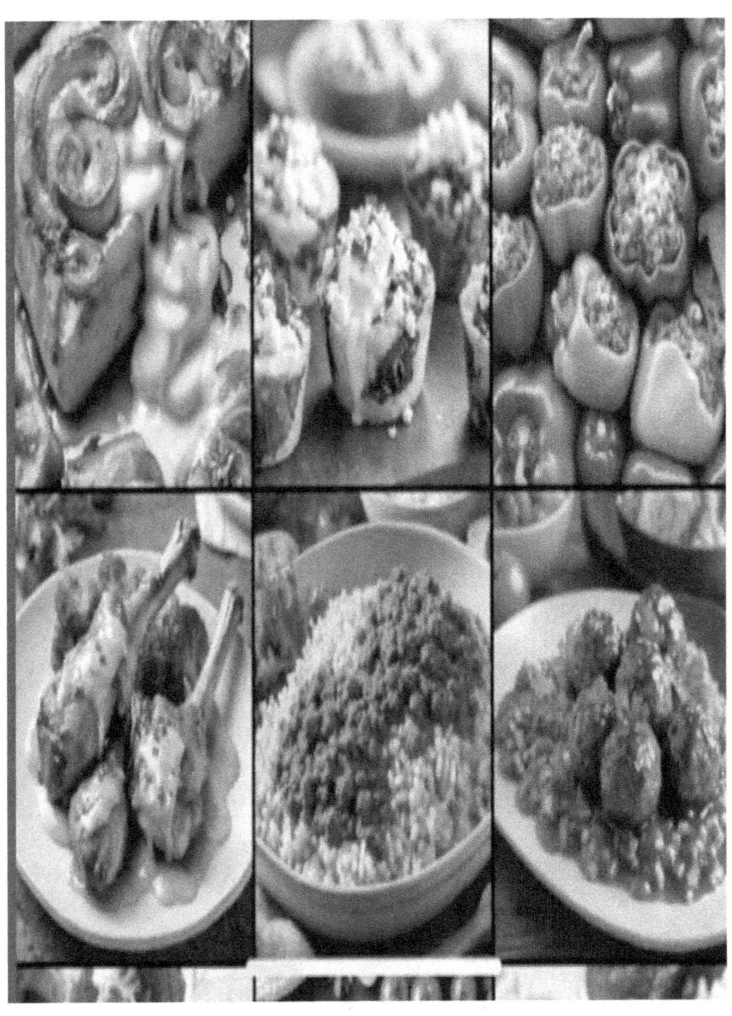

Exploring Global Cuisine for Inspired Combinations

Exploring global cuisine opens a world of culinary possibilities, inviting adventurous food enthusiasts to create inspired combinations that fuse diverse flavors, techniques, and ingredients. From the aromatic spices of Indian cuisine to the umami-rich elements of Japanese dishes, the journey into global gastronomy promises a delightful fusion of traditions.

1. Diverse Influences:

Global cuisine reflects a tapestry of cultural influences, blending regional ingredients and cooking styles. Whether it's the bold flavors of Mexican street food or the delicate balance of Mediterranean dishes, each culinary tradition offers a unique palette for inspired combinations.

2. Ingredients as Storytellers:

Ingredients serve as storytellers, narrating tales of local terroir and culinary heritage. By combining ingredients from different corners of the world, chefs and home cooks alike can weave narratives on their plates, creating dishes that transcend geographical boundaries.

3. Spice Routes and Aromas:

The use of spices defines many global cuisines. Exploring spice routes allows for the creation of intriguing combinations. Imagine the warmth of cumin meeting the citrusy notes of coriander or the subtle heat of chili peppers harmonizing with sweet cinnamon – a symphony of aromas that transcends borders.

4. Fusion Techniques:

Inspired combinations often involve the amalgamation of cooking techniques. Picture the precision of French sous-vide cooking enhancing the tenderness of South American meats, or the artful sushi-making skills from Japan influencing the presentation of a Mediterranean-inspired seafood dish.

5. Cross-Cultural Pairings:

Pairing wines, spirits, or non-alcoholic beverages from different regions complements the culinary experience. The effervescence of champagne with the spiciness of Thai cuisine or the earthiness of red wine with the richness of Italian pasta showcase the potential for delightful cross-cultural pairings.

6. Street Food Inspirations:

Street food, with its authenticity and bold flavors, serves as a rich source of inspiration. From the bustling markets of Marrakech to the vibrant street stalls of Bangkok, incorporating street food elements into your cooking adds a touch of global flair to your creations.

7. Seasonality and Sustainability:

Exploring global cuisine encourages an appreciation for seasonality and sustainability. By incorporating locally sourced, seasonal produce into dishes inspired by different culinary traditions, one can create a harmonious blend of flavors while supporting eco-friendly practices.

8. Culinary Innovation:

Inspired combinations often lead to culinary innovation. Chefs experiment with unexpected pairings, pushing the boundaries of tradition to create novel dishes that captivate the palate and spark a sense of culinary exploration.

In conclusion, exploring global cuisine for inspired combinations is a journey that transcends borders, offering a rich tapestry of flavors, stories, and techniques. It's an opportunity to celebrate the diversity of our world through the universal language of food, inspiring creativity in the kitchen and fostering a deeper appreciation for the culinary traditions that make each culture unique.

CHAPTER 2 :Special Considerations

Special considerations on food combinations involve understanding how different foods interact in the body and impact health. Factors such as nutritional synergy, digestion efficiency, and potential adverse reactions should be taken into account for optimal well-being.

1. Nutritional Synergy:

- Combining complementary nutrients enhances absorption and utilization. For example, pairing vitamin C-rich foods with iron-rich sources improves iron absorption.

- Including healthy fats with vegetables increases the absorption of fat-soluble vitamins like A, D, E, and K.

2. Digestive Compatibility:

- Some foods digest at different rates. Combining fast-digesting fruits with slower-digesting proteins may cause discomfort. Optimal digestion is achieved by pairing foods with similar digestive requirements.

- Avoiding simultaneous consumption of conflicting food groups, like proteins and starches, may ease digestion.

3. Blood Sugar Regulation:

- Balancing carbohydrates with proteins and fats helps regulate blood sugar levels. This prevents rapid spikes and crashes, promoting sustained energy and preventing insulin resistance.

- Fiber-rich foods, like whole grains and vegetables, slow down carbohydrate absorption, aiding blood sugar control.

4. Allergies and Sensitivities:

- Recognizing and avoiding food combinations that trigger allergies or sensitivities is crucial. This includes considering cross-reactivity between allergens.

- Individuals with lactose intolerance may need to be mindful of dairy-containing combinations.

5. Gut Health:

- Probiotic-rich foods (e.g., yogurt, sauerkraut) combined with prebiotic sources (e.g., fiber-rich foods) promote a healthy gut microbiome.

- Limiting highly processed foods and artificial additives supports gut health.

6. Optimal Nutrient Absorption:

- Certain nutrients compete for absorption. Calcium and iron, for instance, may interfere with each other's absorption when consumed simultaneously.

- Proper food timing can enhance nutrient utilization, ensuring maximum benefits from the diet.

7. Cultural and Personal Preferences:

- Cultural traditions and personal preferences play a role in food combinations. Traditional diets often have inherent wisdom in combining foods for taste, nutrition, and digestion.

- Individual dietary choices, such as vegetarian or vegan lifestyles, may require careful planning to ensure nutritional adequacy.

8. Weight Management:

- Balancing macronutrients and considering calorie density can aid in weight management. Combining lean proteins, whole grains, and vegetables promotes satiety and supports weight goals.

- Mindful eating and portion control contribute to overall well-being.

In conclusion, special considerations on food combinations involve a nuanced understanding of nutritional science, individual needs, and cultural factors. Adopting a balanced and varied diet, personalized to one's preferences and requirements, contributes to overall health and vitality.

Food Combinations for Specific Diets (e.g., Vegan, Paleo)

Maintaining a healthy lifestyle often involves adhering to specific diets tailored to individual needs. Understanding optimal food combinations enhances the effectiveness of these diets, ensuring proper nutrition absorption and promoting overall well-being. Here's a comprehensive guide to food combinations for various diets:

1. Ketogenic Diet:

   - Combine healthy fats with moderate protein and minimal carbs.

   - Pair avocados with lean meats or fatty fish.

- Opt for olive oil-based dressings on protein-rich salads.

2. Paleo Diet:

- Focus on whole foods, emphasizing lean meats, fruits, and vegetables.

- Combine lean protein sources with colorful veggies.

- Include nuts and seeds for added nutrients.

3. Vegetarian/Vegan Diet:

- Combine complementary plant proteins, such as beans and rice.

- Pair iron-rich foods with vitamin C sources for better absorption.

- Incorporate nuts and seeds for essential fats and proteins.

4. Mediterranean Diet:

- Combine olive oil with vegetables for a rich source of healthy fats.

- Pair fish with whole grains like quinoa or brown rice.

- Include a variety of colorful fruits and vegetables for diverse nutrients.

5. Gluten-Free Diet:

- Choose gluten-free grains like rice, quinoa, or buckwheat.

- Combine lean proteins with gluten-free whole grains.

- Opt for fresh fruits and vegetables as snacks.

6. Low-FODMAP Diet:

- Combine low-FODMAP fruits and vegetables with tolerated proteins.

- Avoid high-FODMAP combinations like certain legumes and grains.

- Experiment with suitable herbs and spices for flavor.

7. DASH Diet (for Hypertension):

- Combine potassium-rich foods (bananas, oranges) with low-sodium options.

- Pair lean proteins with whole grains and vegetables.

- Use herbs and spices instead of excessive salt for flavor.

8. Blood Type Diet:

- Tailor food combinations based on individual blood type recommendations.

- Emphasize lean proteins, fruits, and vegetables specific to your blood type.

- Monitor energy levels and digestion for personalized adjustments.

9. Intermittent Fasting:

- Focus on nutrient-dense meals during eating windows.

- Combine proteins, healthy fats, and fiber for sustained energy.

- Stay hydrated during fasting periods with water, herbal tea, or black coffee.

10. Heart-Healthy Diet:

- Pair omega-3 fatty acid-rich fish with whole grains and vegetables.

- Choose lean proteins and incorporate sources of soluble fiber.

- Limit saturated and trans fats by opting for healthier cooking methods.

Remember, individual responses to diets can vary, so it's crucial to listen to your body and consult with a healthcare professional or nutritionist for personalized advice.

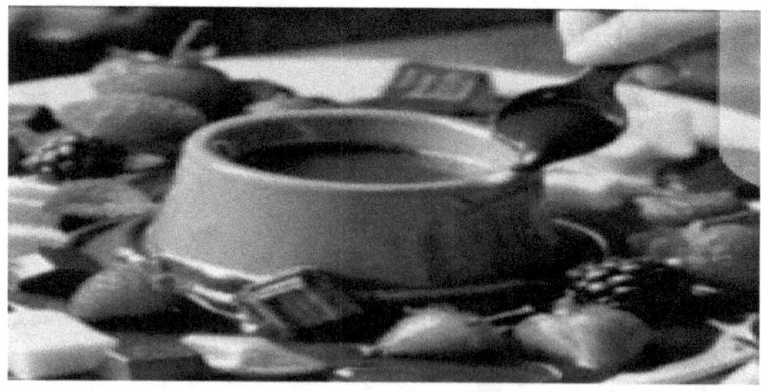

Tailoring Combinations for Dietary Restrictions

Tailoring combinations for dietary restrictions involves creating meal plans that accommodate specific dietary needs, ensuring individuals can enjoy a well-balanced and nutritionally adequate diet. Here's a comprehensive guide to tailoring combinations for various dietary restrictions:

1. Understanding Dietary Restrictions:

- Identify specific dietary restrictions such as allergies, intolerances, or lifestyle choices like vegetarianism or veganism.

- Consider medical conditions like celiac disease, diabetes, or hypertension that may require specific dietary adjustments.

2. Creating a Balanced Plate:

- Focus on a variety of whole foods, including fruits, vegetables, lean proteins, whole grains, and healthy fats.

- Ensure meals are well-balanced with a mix of macronutrients (carbohydrates, proteins, and fats) and micronutrients (vitamins and minerals).

3. Allergies and Intolerances:

- Exclude allergens or intolerant foods while substituting with alternatives.

- Read food labels carefully to avoid hidden allergens.

4. Vegetarian and Vegan Combinations:

- Incorporate plant-based protein sources such as beans, lentils, tofu, and tempeh.

- Ensure a variety of colorful vegetables and fruits to meet nutritional needs.

5. Gluten-Free Options:

- Choose gluten-free grains like quinoa, rice, and corn.

- Use gluten-free flour alternatives for baking.

6. Diabetic-Friendly Choices:

- Opt for complex carbohydrates with a low glycemic index.

- Include lean proteins and healthy fats to stabilize blood sugar levels.

7. Heart-Healthy Meals:

- Focus on lean proteins, whole grains, and foods rich in omega-3 fatty acids.

- Limit saturated fats and sodium intake.

8. Renal Diet Considerations:

- Monitor phosphorus, potassium, and sodium intake.

- Choose foods with lower protein content.

9. Customizing Portion Sizes:

- Adjust portion sizes based on individual caloric needs and goals.

- Use smaller, more frequent meals to manage energy levels.

10. Meal Prep and Planning:

- Plan meals in advance to ensure a variety of nutrients.

- Batch cook and store meals for convenience.

11. Seeking Professional Guidance:

- Consult with a registered dietitian or nutritionist for personalized advice.

- Consider professional support for complex dietary needs or medical conditions.

12. Emphasizing Flavor and Variety:

- Experiment with herbs, spices, and different cooking techniques to enhance flavors.

- Include a wide array of foods to prevent monotony.

Tailoring combinations for dietary restrictions involves a thoughtful and informed approach, considering individual preferences and nutritional requirements. It's essential to maintain a well-rounded diet that promotes overall health while adhering to specific dietary constraints.

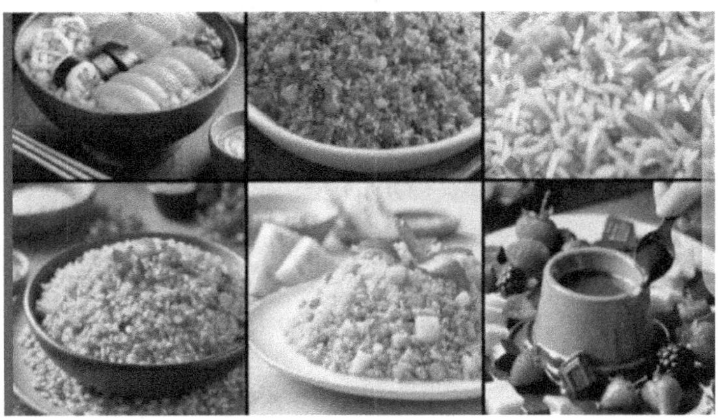

CHAPTER 3 :Digestive Health

Digestive health plays a crucial role in our overall well-being, influencing nutrient absorption, immune function, and even mental health. One approach to enhance digestive health is through mindful food combining, a practice rooted in optimizing nutrient absorption and reducing digestive discomfort.

Understanding Food Combining:

Food combining involves pairing foods based on their compatibility in terms of digestion. The premise is that certain food combinations may ease the digestive process, promoting efficient nutrient absorption and minimizing digestive issues.

Principles of Food Combining:

1. Separating Protein and Starches: Consuming proteins and starches separately can aid digestion. This is based on the idea that different enzymes are required for the digestion of these macronutrients.

2. Fruit Consumption Alone: Fruits are typically recommended to be eaten alone or on an empty stomach. This is due to their quick digestion time, preventing fermentation and potential discomfort when mixed with slower-digesting foods.

3. Avoiding Mixing Certain Food Groups: Some food combining philosophies suggest avoiding combining certain food groups, such as proteins and acidic fruits or starches with acidic foods, to prevent potential digestive conflicts.

Benefits of Food Combining for Digestive Health:

1. Reduced Bloating and Gas: Proper food combining may help alleviate common digestive issues like bloating and gas by optimizing the digestion process.

2. Enhanced Nutrient Absorption: By aligning food combinations with optimal digestion, the body may absorb nutrients more effectively, supporting overall health and vitality.

3. Improved Energy Levels: Digestive efficiency contributes to increased energy levels as the body can use nutrients more efficiently for various physiological processes.

Sample Food Combining Guidelines:

1. Separate Proteins and Starches: For example, avoid combining meat and potatoes in the same meal.

2. Consume Fruits Alone: Eat fruits on an empty stomach or as a snack between meals.

3. Mindful Pairing: Pairing vegetables with either proteins or starches is often considered a balanced approach.

Considerations and Criticisms:

While some individuals report benefits from food combining, it's essential to note that scientific evidence supporting these practices is limited. Nutrient absorption is a complex process influenced by various factors beyond food combinationsn

Conclusion:

Prioritizing digestive health through mindful food combining can be a personal choice. It's crucial to listen to your body, observe how it responds to different food combinations, and consult with healthcare professionals for personalized advice. While food combining might offer benefits for some, it's essential to maintain a balanced and varied diet for overall well-being.

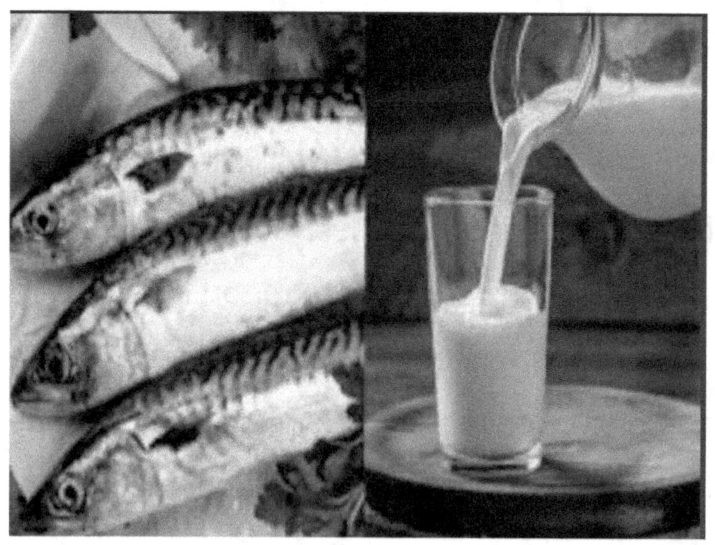

Digestive health is crucial for overall well-being, as it plays a fundamental role in nutrient absorption, immune function, and waste elimination. Several key components contribute to maintaining optimal digestive health.

1. Balanced Diet:

- Include a variety of fruits, vegetables, whole grains, and lean proteins in your diet.

- Fiber-rich foods promote regular bowel movements and support a healthy gut microbiome.

2. Hydration:

- Drink an adequate amount of water to help digest food and prevent constipation.

3. Probiotics:

- Incorporate probiotic-rich foods like yogurt, kefir, sauerkraut, and kimchi to support a diverse and beneficial gut microbiome.

4. Prebiotics:

- Consume prebiotic-rich foods such as garlic, onions, bananas, and asparagus to nourish the growth of beneficial bacteria.

5. Limit Processed Foods:

- Reduce intake of processed and high-sugar foods, as they may negatively impact gut health.

6. Chew Food Thoroughly:

- Chewing food well aids in the digestion process and nutrient absorption in the stomach.

7. Regular Physical Activity:

- Exercise supports healthy digestion by promoting regular bowel movements and reducing the risk of constipation.

8. Manage Stress:

- Chronic stress can affect digestion. Practice stress-reduction techniques such as meditation, deep breathing, or yoga.

9. Adequate Sleep:

- Lack of sleep may disrupt digestive processes. Aim for 7-9 hours of quality sleep per night.

10. Identify Food Intolerances:

- Pay attention to how your body reacts to certain foods and identify any intolerances or sensitivities.

11. Regular Medical Check-ups:

- Consult with healthcare professionals for routine check-ups and address any digestive concerns promptly.

12. Avoid Overeating:

- Practice portion control to prevent overloading the digestive system.

13. Maintain a Healthy Weight:

- Obesity can contribute to digestive issues. Achieve and maintain a healthy weight through balanced nutrition and regular exercise.

14. Limit Alcohol and Caffeine:

- Excessive alcohol and caffeine intake can irritate the digestive tract. Consume them in moderation.

15. Stay Informed:

- Stay informed about digestive health conditions and symptoms. Seek medical advice if you experience persistent issues.

In conclusion, prioritizing digestive health involves a holistic approach encompassing nutrition, lifestyle, and mindfulness. By adopting these habits, individuals can cultivate a resilient digestive system, promoting overall health and vitality.

Promoting Gut Health through Smart Food Choices

Promoting gut health through smart food choices is essential for overall well-being. A balanced and diverse diet plays a pivotal role in maintaining a healthy gut microbiome, which is crucial for digestion, nutrient absorption, and immune function.

1. Include Probiotics:

Incorporating probiotic-rich foods like yogurt, kefir, sauerkraut, and kimchi can introduce beneficial bacteria into the gut. These probiotics help maintain a harmonious balance in the microbiome, promoting digestive health.

2. Fiber-Rich Foods:

Fiber is a key component for gut health, promoting regular bowel movements and providing nourishment for beneficial gut bacteria. Whole grains, fruits, vegetables, and legumes are excellent sources of dietary fiber.

3. Prebiotic Foods:

Include prebiotic-rich foods such as garlic, onions, leeks, bananas, and asparagus. Prebiotics are non-digestible fibers that serve as food for beneficial gut bacteria, fostering their growth and activity.

4. Variety of Fruits and Vegetables:

Consuming a diverse range of fruits and vegetables ensures a broad spectrum of nutrients and phytochemicals, which can positively impact gut health. Different plant compounds support various aspects of digestive function.

5. Limit Processed Foods:

Processed foods often contain additives and preservatives that may negatively impact the gut microbiome. Opt for whole, unprocessed foods to promote a healthier balance of gut bacteria.

6. Stay Hydrated:

Adequate water intake is vital for digestion and overall gut health. Water helps maintain the mucosal lining of the intestines, facilitating smooth passage of food and nutrients.

7. Include Omega-3 Fatty Acids:

Omega-3 fatty acids, found in fatty fish, flaxseeds, and walnuts, have anti-inflammatory properties that can benefit the gut. Chronic inflammation is linked to various gastrointestinal issues, so including omega-3s can support gut health.

8. Limit Artificial Sweeteners:

Some artificial sweeteners may alter the composition of the gut microbiome. Consider reducing the intake of these sweeteners to maintain a healthy balance of gut bacteria.

9. Manage Stress:

Stress can impact gut health, and vice versa. Incorporate stress-management techniques such as meditation, yoga, or deep breathing exercises to promote a healthy gut-brain connection.

10. Personalized Approach:

Recognize that individual responses to food can vary. Experiment with different foods and monitor how your body reacts. A personalized approach to nutrition can help identify foods that specifically benefit your gut health.

By making informed and mindful food choices, you can cultivate a thriving gut microbiome, leading to improved digestion, nutrient absorption, and overall well-being.

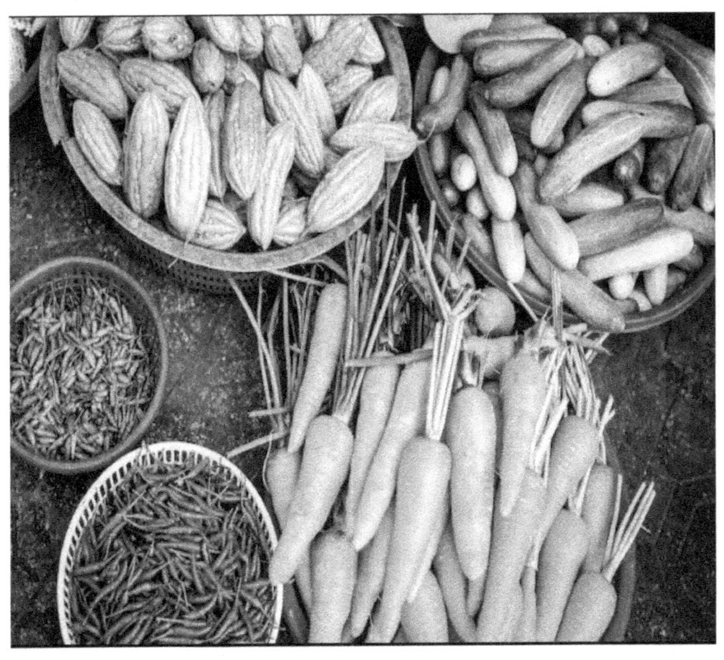

Foods that Aid Digestion

Proper digestion is crucial for overall health, and incorporating foods that aid digestion into your diet can promote a well-functioning digestive system. Here's a comprehensive guide to such foods:

1. Fiber-Rich Foods:

- **Benefits**: Enhances bowel regularity and prevents constipation.

- **Examples**: Whole grains, fruits, vegetables, legumes, and nuts.

2. Probiotics:

- *Benefits:* Promotes a healthy balance of gut bacteria, aiding in digestion.

- *Examples:* Yogurt, kefir, sauerkraut, kimchi, and other fermented foods.

3. Ginger:

- **Benefits**: Alleviates digestive discomfort, reduces nausea, and stimulates saliva production.

- **Usage**: Add fresh ginger to teas, smoothies, or include it in cooking.

4. Peppermint:

- **Benefits**: Relaxes muscles in the gastrointestinal tract, easing indigestion.

- **Usage**: Peppermint tea or adding fresh peppermint leaves to meals.

5. Papaya:

- **Benefits**: Contains enzymes like papain, aiding in protein digestion.

- **Usage**: Eat ripe papaya as a snack or incorporate it into salads.

6. Fennel:

- **Benefits**: Eases bloating and gas, relaxes the digestive tract.

- **Usage**: Chew on fennel seeds or add sliced fennel to salads.

7. Bananas:

- **Benefits**: Non-acidic and easily digestible, soothing for the stomach.

- Usage: Enjoy as a snack or add to smoothies.

8. Whole Grains:

- **Benefits**: Provide essential nutrients and fiber, supporting regular bowel movements.

- **Examples**: Brown rice, quinoa, oats, and whole wheat.

9. Lean Proteins:

- **Benefits**: Easier to digest compared to fatty meats.

- **Examples**: Skinless poultry, fish, tofu, and legumes.

10. Water:

- **Benefits**: Maintains hydration, aids in the softening and movement of stool.

- **Usage**: Drink an adequate amount throughout the day.

11. Turmeric:

- *Benefits:* Possesses anti-inflammatory properties, aids digestion.

- **Usage**: Add turmeric to curries, soups, or make turmeric tea.

12. Chamomile Tea:

- **Benefits**: Calms the digestive tract, relieves indigestion and gas.

- **Usage**: Drink chamomile tea after meals.

13. Lemon Water:

- **Benefits**: Stimulates digestive enzymes and provides vitamin C.

- **Usage**: Squeeze fresh lemon into water and drink before meals.

14. Avocado:

- **Benefits**: Contains healthy fats that support nutrient absorption.

- **Usage**: Include sliced avocado in salads or as a topping.

15. Cinnamon:

- **Benefits**: Aids in digestion, may help alleviate bloating.

- **Usage**: Sprinkle cinnamon on oatmeal, yogurt, or in beverages.

Incorporating a variety of these foods into your diet can contribute to a well-balanced and digestion-friendly eating plan. Remember to listen to your body and make adjustments based on your individual needs.

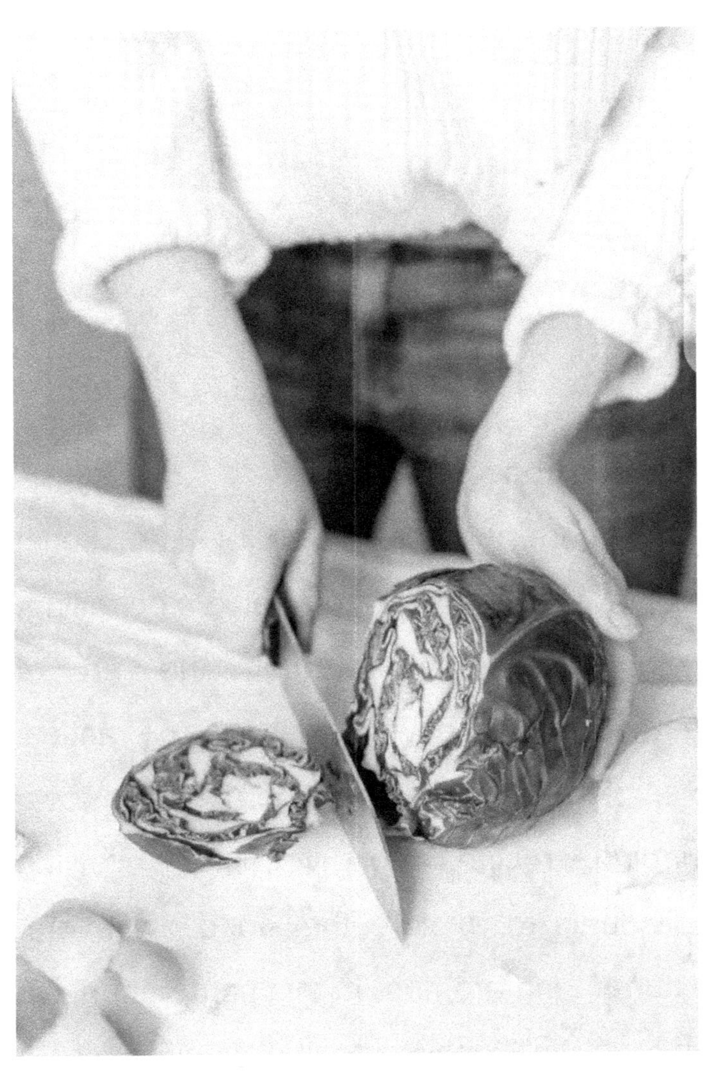

CHAPTER 4: Recipes and Practical Examples

Introduction

Recipes are not merely a set of instructions; they are a form of culinary storytelling, guiding individuals through the art of creating delightful dishes. Practical examples serve as hands-on experiences, bringing recipes to life and allowing individuals to explore the world of flavors, textures, and aromas. In this comprehensive content, we'll delve into the significance of recipes, their structure, and the importance of practical examples in mastering the culinary arts.

The Art of Recipes

Structure of a Recipe

A well-crafted recipe is like a carefully composed symphony, with each ingredient and step contributing to the overall harmony. Key components of a recipe include:

1. **Ingredients**: The building blocks of a dish. Clearly list the quantities and types of ingredients needed.

2. **PInstructions**: Step-by-step guidance on how to combine and prepare the ingredients. Clarity and precision are crucial to ensure a successful outcome.

3. **Cooking Time and Temperature**: Specify the duration and temperature for

cooking or baking. This information is vital for achieving the desired taste and texture.

4. Servings: Indicate the number of servings the recipe yields. This helps individuals plan accordingly.

Adaptability of Recipes

Recipes are versatile and can be adapted to suit individual preferences, dietary restrictions, or ingredient availability. Encouraging experimentation fosters creativity and allows cooks to put their unique twist on traditional dishes.

Practical Examples in Culinary Learning

Hands-On Learning

Practical examples provide a tangible experience that complements theoretical knowledge. Cooking is an art best learned through practice, and practical examples offer the opportunity for individuals to hone their skills in a real kitchen environment.

Skill Development

From knife skills to mastering different cooking techniques, practical examples play a crucial role in skill development. Through hands-on experiences, individuals gain confidence in handling ingredients, understanding flavor profiles, and executing intricate cooking methods.

Problem-Solving

Cooking is not without challenges. Practical examples present opportunities to troubleshoot common issues such as overcooking, under-seasoning, or adjusting the consistency of a dish. These challenges enhance problem-solving skills and resilience in the kitchen.

Examples of Recipes with Practical Application

1. Classic Spaghetti Bolognese:

- **Ingredients**: Ground beef, onions, garlic, tomatoes, pasta.

- **Practical Example**: Browning meat, sautéing aromatics, and mastering the perfect al dente pasta.

2. Homemade Pizza:

- **Ingredients**: Pizza dough, tomato sauce, cheese, toppings of choice.

- **Practical Example**: Kneading dough, spreading sauce, and creating personalized pizza combinations.

3. Vegetable Stir-Fry:

- **Ingredients:** Assorted vegetables, soy sauce, ginger, garlic.

- **Practical Example**: Quick cooking, maintaining crispness, and achieving a balanced stir-fry sauce.

Conclusion

Recipes and practical examples are integral components of culinary education. They not only guide individuals in creating delicious meals but also empower them to become confident, creative cooks. Whether following a traditional recipe or putting a unique spin on a classic dish, the combination of structured guidance and hands-on experience is the recipe for culinary success.

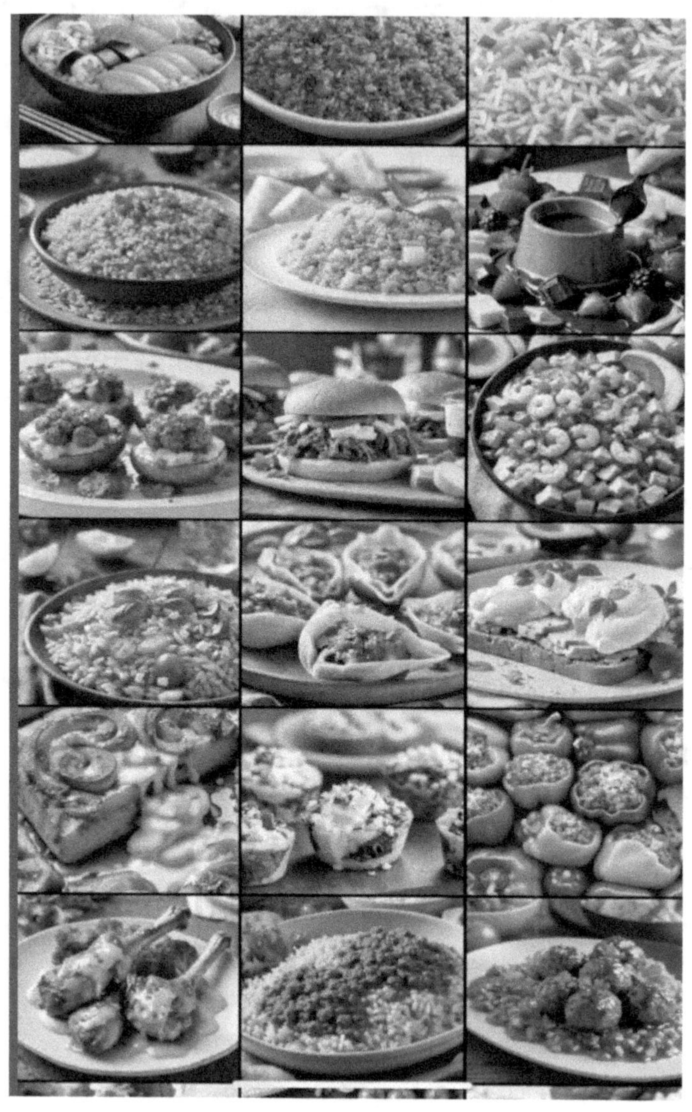

Breakfast Ideas for Delicious Food Combinations

Breakfast is the most important meal of the day, and what better way to start your morning than with a flavorful and satisfying combination of foods? Here are some creative and nutritious breakfast ideas that combine various ingredients to kickstart your day:

1. Avocado Toast with Poached Egg:

- Spread ripe avocado on whole-grain toast and top it with a perfectly poached egg. The creamy avocado complements the runny yolk, creating a harmonious blend of textures.

2. Greek Yogurt Parfait:

- Layer Greek yogurt with granola, fresh berries, and a drizzle of honey. This parfait provides a balance of protein, fiber, and natural sweetness, making it both delicious and nutritious.

3. Oatmeal with Nut Butter and Banana Slices:

- Enhance your oatmeal by stirring in almond or peanut butter and adding banana slices. The combination of hearty oats, creamy nut butter, and sweet bananas creates a wholesome and filling breakfast.

4. Smoked Salmon Bagel with Cream Cheese:

- Enjoy a classic combination of smoked salmon and cream cheese on a toasted bagel. The richness of the cream cheese complements the smoky flavor of the salmon, creating a luxurious and satisfying meal.

5. Veggie Omelette with Whole Wheat Toast:

- Whisk eggs and fill your omelette with a variety of colorful vegetables such as bell peppers, spinach, and tomatoes. Pair it with whole wheat toast for a well-rounded breakfast that provides protein and complex carbohydrates.

6. Chia Seed Pudding with Fresh Fruit:

- Mix chia seeds with milk or a plant-based alternative and let it sit overnight. Top the pudding with fresh fruit like berries, mango, or kiwi for a delightful and nutritious breakfast bowl.

7. Banana Pancakes with Maple Syrup and Nuts:

- Make fluffy banana pancakes and drizzle them with pure maple syrup. Sprinkle chopped nuts like walnuts or almonds for added crunch and a boost of healthy fats.

8. Smoothie Bowl with Toppings:

- Blend your favorite fruits, leafy greens, and yogurt into a smoothie, then pour it into a bowl. Top it with granola, chia seeds, and sliced fruits for a vibrant and satisfying breakfast bowl.

9. Whole Grain Waffles with Berries and Whipped Cream:

- Opt for whole grain waffles topped with a mix of fresh berries and a dollop of whipped cream. This delightful combination adds sweetness and a touch of indulgence to your morning.

10. Breakfast Burrito with Avocado and Salsa:

- Fill a whole-grain tortilla with scrambled eggs, black beans, avocado slices, and salsa. This savory breakfast burrito provides a burst of flavors and a good balance of protein and fiber.

Experiment with these breakfast combinations to discover your favorite morning fuel. Remember to customize portion sizes based on your dietary needs and preferences

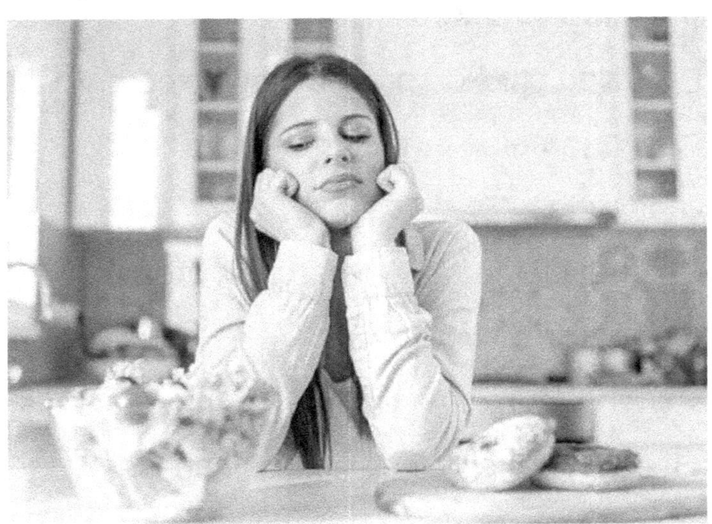

Lunch and Dinner Combinations

Sure, here are some lunch and dinner combinations that offer a mix of flavors, nutrients, and satisfaction:

Lunch Combinations:

1. Grilled Chicken Salad:

- Grilled chicken breast with mixed greens, cherry tomatoes, cucumbers, and a light vinaigrette.

- Side: Quinoa or whole-grain bread.

2. Vegetarian Wrap:

- Whole-grain wrap filled with hummus, roasted vegetables, feta cheese, and spinach.

- Side: Fresh fruit or a side salad.

3. Tuna and Avocado Sandwich:

- Tuna salad made with light mayo, mixed with diced avocado on whole-grain bread.

- Side: Baked sweet potato fries or a handful of nuts.

4. Mediterranean Bowl:

- Quinoa base topped with cherry tomatoes, olives, feta cheese, roasted chickpeas, and a drizzle of olive oil.

- Side: Greek yogurt with honey.

Dinner Combinations:

1. Salmon with Roasted Vegetables:

- Baked or grilled salmon with a side of roasted Brussels sprouts, carrots, and sweet potatoes.

- Side: Quinoa or brown rice.

2. Stir-Fried Tofu and Vegetables:

  - Tofu stir-fried with a colorful mix of broccoli, bell peppers, and snap peas in a light soy-ginger sauce.

  - Side: Brown rice or cauliflower rice.

3. Spaghetti Bolognese:

  - Whole-grain or lentil-based spaghetti with a lean ground turkey or beef Bolognese sauce.

  - Side: Mixed green salad.

4. Chickpea Curry:

  - Chickpeas simmered in a flavorful curry sauce with tomatoes, onions, and spices.

  - Side: Quinoa or basmati rice.

 General Tips:

- **Incorporate Color**: Include a variety of colorful vegetables to ensure a diverse range of nutrients.

- **Lean Proteins**: Opt for lean protein sources like chicken, fish, tofu, or legumes.

- **Whole Grains**: Choose whole grains like quinoa, brown rice, or whole-grain bread for added fiber and nutrients.

- **Balanced Plates**: Aim for a balance of carbohydrates, proteins, and healthy fats in each meal.

- **Portion Control**: Be mindful of portion sizes to maintain a balanced and healthy diet.

Remember to customize these combinations based on personal preferences and dietary needs.

Snack Options

Snacking can be both delightful and nutritious when you explore a variety of food combinations. Consider these options for a satisfying snack experience:

1. Hummus and Veggie Sticks:

   - Pair creamy hummus with colorful carrot, cucumber, and bell pepper sticks for a crunchy and protein-packed snack.

2. Greek Yogurt Parfait:

   - Layer Greek yogurt with granola, fresh berries, and a drizzle of honey for a balanced mix of protein, fiber, and vitamins.

3. Avocado Toast:

   - Spread ripe avocado on whole-grain toast and sprinkle with a pinch of sea salt and red pepper flakes for a tasty combination of healthy fats and carbohydrates.

4. Cheese and Whole Grain Crackers:

- Enjoy a satisfying blend of protein and whole grains by pairing your favorite cheese with whole grain crackers or rice cakes.

5. Trail Mix:

- Create a customized trail mix with a mix of nuts, seeds, dried fruits, and a touch of dark chocolate for a convenient and energy-boosting snack.

6. Apple Slices with Nut Butter:

- Slice up a crisp apple and dip it in almond or peanut butter for a delicious combination of natural sweetness and protein.

7. Caprese Skewers:

- Thread cherry tomatoes, fresh mozzarella, and basil leaves onto skewers, then drizzle with balsamic glaze for a refreshing and savory snack.

8. Popcorn with Nutritional Yeast:

- Sprinkle air-popped popcorn with nutritional yeast for a savory, cheesy flavor without the extra calories, creating a satisfying whole-grain snack.

9. Rice Cake Pizzas:

- Top rice cakes with tomato sauce, mozzarella, and your favorite pizza toppings for a lighter twist on the classic pizza.

10. Edamame:

- Boil or steam edamame and lightly salt them for a protein-rich and satisfying snack that's also rich in fiber.

11. Cottage Cheese with Pineapple:

- Combine cottage cheese with fresh pineapple chunks for a sweet and tangy snack that provides a good balance of protein and vitamins.

12. Dark Chocolate and Almonds:

- Pair a few squares of dark chocolate with almonds for a delightful mix of antioxidants, healthy fats, and a satisfying crunch.

Remember to stay mindful of portion sizes and opt for whole, minimally processed ingredients to maximize nutritional benefits while enjoying your snack combinations.

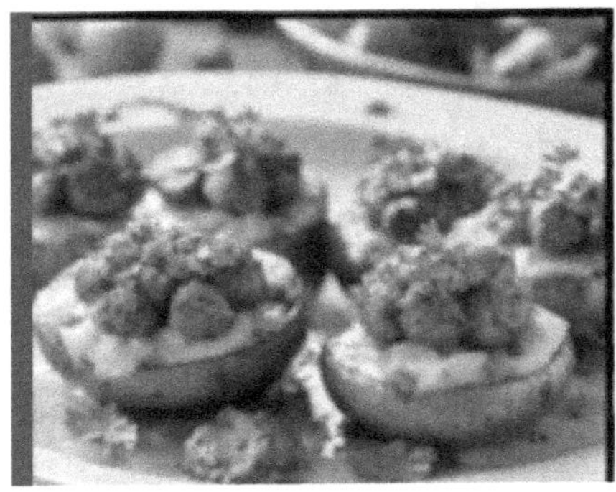

CHAPTER 5:Summary of Key Principle

Eating a well-balanced and nutritious diet involves not only choosing the right foods but also considering how these foods are combined. The principles of food combinations play a crucial role in optimizing digestion, nutrient absorption, and overall health. Here's a comprehensive summary of key principles for effective food combinations:

1. Protein and Starch Separation:

- Avoid combining high-protein foods with high-starch foods in the same meal.

- Proteins require an acidic environment for digestion, while starches need an alkaline environment. Combining both may lead to inefficient digestion.

2. Fruits on an Empty Stomach:

- Consume fruits separately from other foods and preferably on an empty stomach.

- Fruits digest quickly, and when eaten alone, they prevent fermentation and potential digestive issues.

3. Protein and Non-Starchy Vegetables:

- Pairing proteins with non-starchy vegetables is generally well-tolerated and supports optimal digestion.

- Non-starchy vegetables provide essential nutrients and fiber without interfering with protein digestion.

4. Fats with Non-Starchy Vegetables:

- Combine healthy fats with non-starchy vegetables for better absorption of fat-soluble vitamins.

- Fats slow down the digestion process, allowing for a steady release of nutrients.

5. Limiting Complex Combinations:

- Minimize complex food combinations in one meal to prevent overloading the digestive system.

- Simpler meals are often easier for the body to process, leading to improved nutrient absorption.

6. Acidic and Alkaline Foods:

- Balance acidic and alkaline foods in your diet for optimal pH levels in the body.

- Including a variety of fruits, vegetables, and whole grains helps maintain a healthy acid-alkaline balance.

7. Hydration Timing:

- Avoid drinking large amounts of liquids during meals as it can dilute digestive enzymes.

- Stay hydrated between meals to support overall bodily functions.

8. Mindful Eating:

- Practice mindful eating by savoring each bite and paying attention to hunger and fullness cues.

- Chew food thoroughly to aid in digestion and nutrient absorption.

9. Personalized Approach:

- Consider individual differences in digestion and tolerance.

- Some individuals may have specific sensitivities or preferences, so adjust food combinations based on personal needs.

10. Experiment and Observe:

- Pay attention to how your body responds to different food combinations.

- Experiment with variations and observe energy levels, digestion, and overall well-being.

Incorporating these principles into your dietary habits can contribute to improved digestion, nutrient utilization, and overall health. Remember that individual needs vary, so it's essential to find a balance that works best for you.

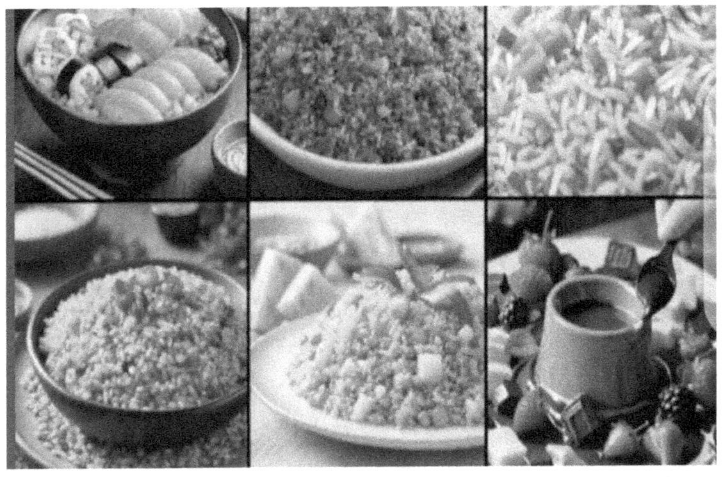

Incorporating Food Combinations into Daily Life

Incorporating food combinations into your daily life is a key aspect of maintaining a well-balanced and nutritious diet. By strategically pairing different food groups, you can enhance nutrient absorption, improve digestion, and even optimize energy levels. Here's a comprehensive guide to help you make informed choices:

1. Balanced Meals:

   - Aim for a combination of macronutrients in each meal—protein, carbohydrates, and healthy fats. This ensures sustained energy and overall nutritional completeness.

2. Protein and Fiber Pairing:

   - Combine lean proteins like chicken, fish, or legumes with high-fiber foods such as vegetables, whole grains, or fruits. This not only promotes satiety but also supports digestive health.

3. Nutrient Synergy:

   - Pairing certain foods enhances nutrient absorption. For instance, consuming vitamin C-rich foods with iron sources increases iron absorption. Examples include spinach with citrus fruits or bell peppers with beans.

4. Healthy Fats with Greens:

   - Incorporate healthy fats like avocados, nuts, or olive oil with leafy greens. Fats aid in the absorption of fat-soluble vitamins present in vegetables, making the nutrients more bioavailable.

5. Cautious Carbohydrate Combining:

- Be mindful of carbohydrate combinations. Pairing complex carbohydrates with lean proteins or healthy fats can help stabilize blood sugar levels. Examples include brown rice with grilled chicken or quinoa with vegetables.

6. Dairy and Magnesium:

- Dairy products are rich in calcium but can inhibit magnesium absorption. Pairing dairy with magnesium-rich foods like leafy greens, nuts, or seeds ensures a more balanced intake of these essential minerals.

7. Mindful Snacking:

- Opt for nutrient-dense snacks that combine protein, fiber, and healthy fats. Greek yogurt with berries, apple slices with almond butter, or hummus with carrot sticks are excellent choices.

8. Hydration and Nutrient Absorption:

- Stay hydrated to support digestion and nutrient absorption. Water aids in breaking down food particles and transporting nutrients throughout the body.

9. Anti-Inflammatory Combinations:

- Emphasize anti-inflammatory foods by combining fatty fish with colorful vegetables and herbs. This can contribute to reducing inflammation and promoting overall well-being.

10. Customizing for Dietary Needs:

- Consider individual dietary preferences and restrictions. Whether you follow a vegetarian, vegan, or specific dietary plan, tailor food combinations to meet your nutritional requirements.

11. Experiment and Enjoy:

- Explore different food pairings to keep your meals interesting and enjoyable. Trying new combinations ensures a diverse intake of nutrients and prevents dietary monotony. Incorporating thoughtfully paired food combinations into your daily life not only supports your nutritional goals but also contributes to overall health and well-being. Remember to consult with a healthcare professional or nutritionist for personalized advice based on your specific needs and health conditions.

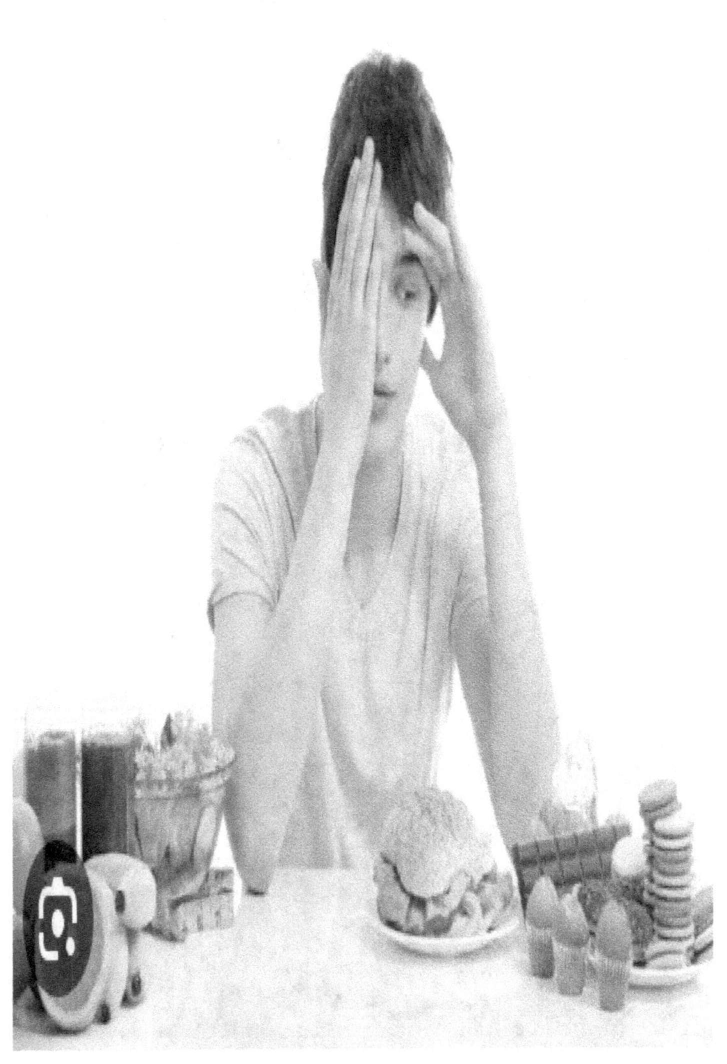

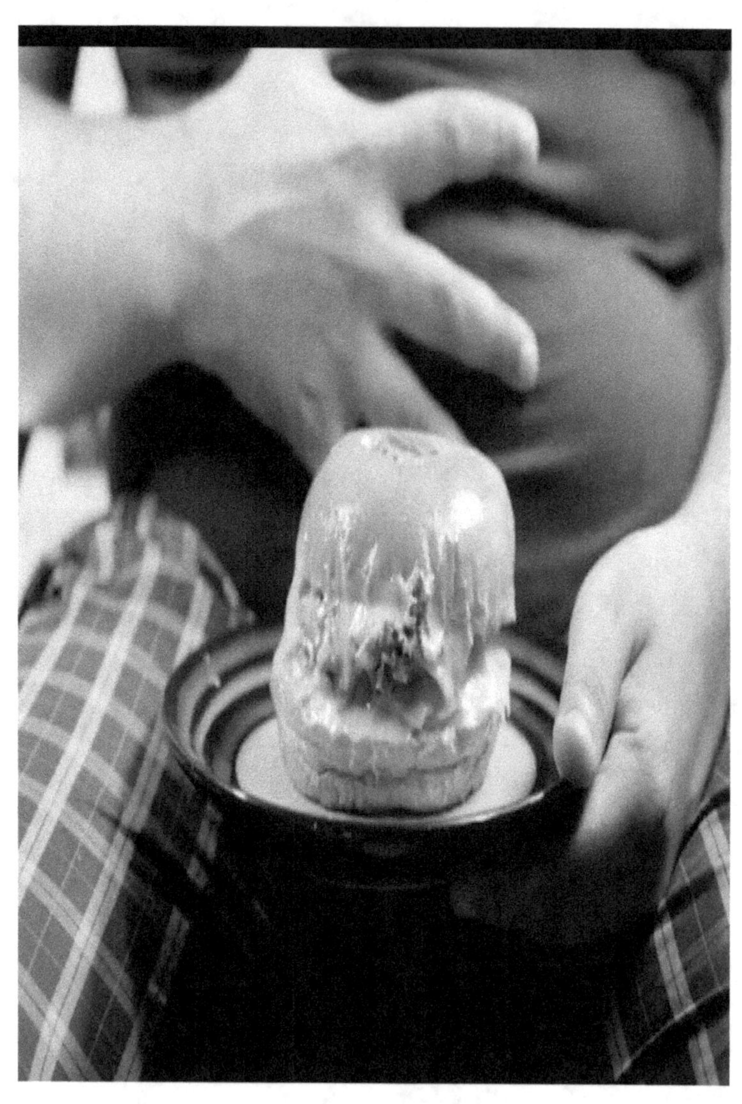

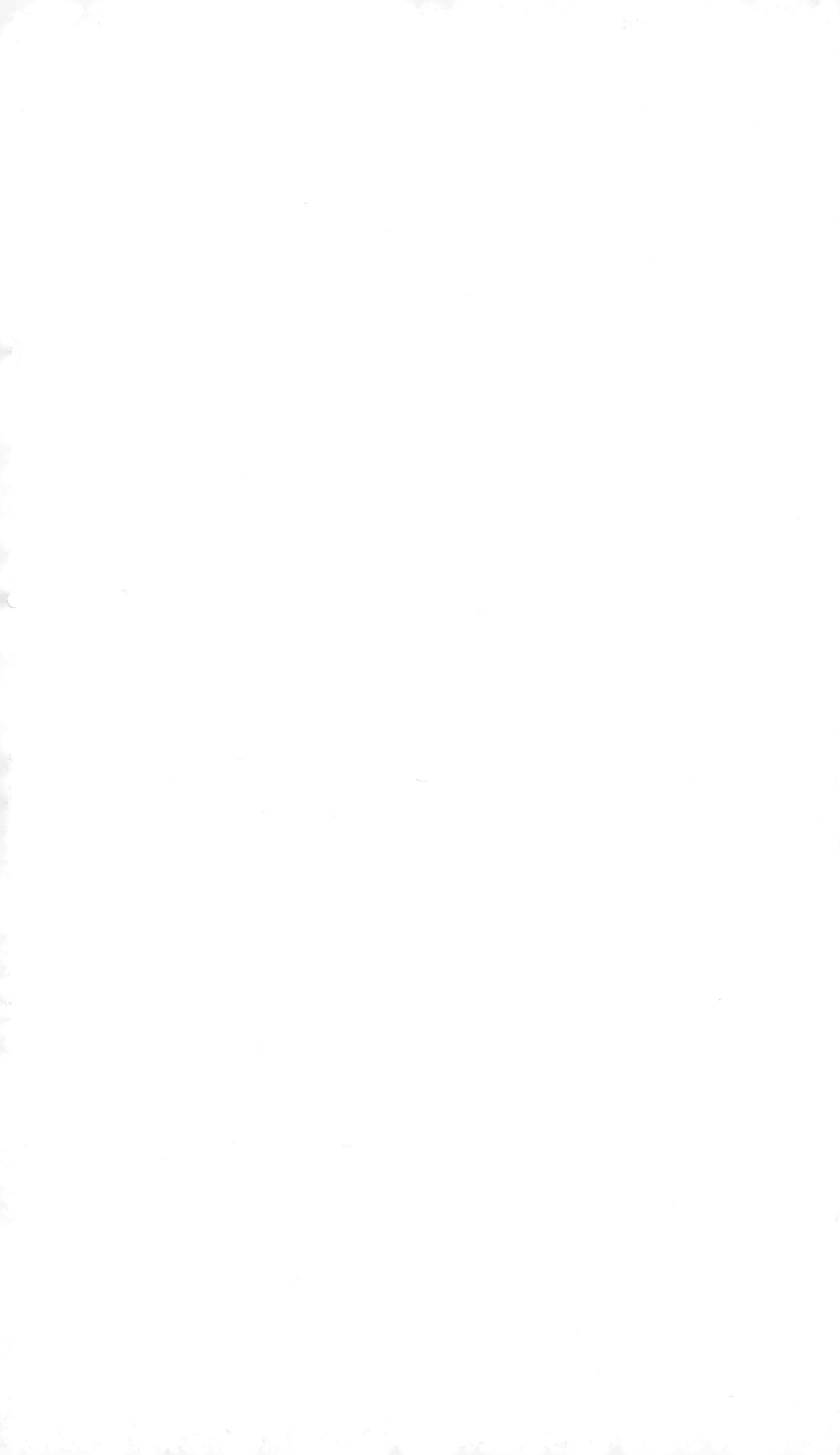